HEALTH, STRENGTH & WILL-POWER

by

MAXICK

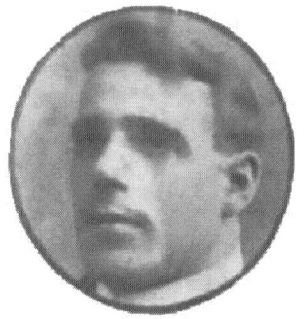

And

SALDO

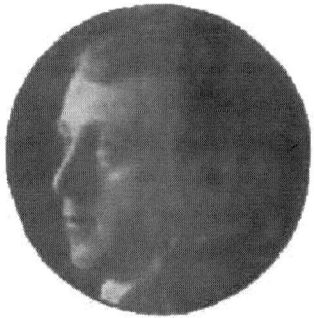

"The city worker would do well to regard the question of health as a question of capital and income."

-Dr. Murray Leslie

DISCLAIMER

The exercises and advice contained within this book is for educational and entertainment purposes only. The exercises described may be too strenuous or dangerous for some people, and the reader should consult with a physician before engaging in any of them.

The author and publisher of this book are not responsible in any manner whatsoever for any injury, which may occur through the use or misuse of the information presented here.

Health, Strength & Will Power originally published in 1911
Modern Reprint Edition

Copyright © 2011 by StrongmanBooks.com
All Rights Reserved.

No part of this course may be reproduced or transmitted in any form or by any means, electronic or mechanical, including photocopying, recording, or by any information storage and retrieval system, without permission in writing from the publisher.

Manufactured in the United States of America

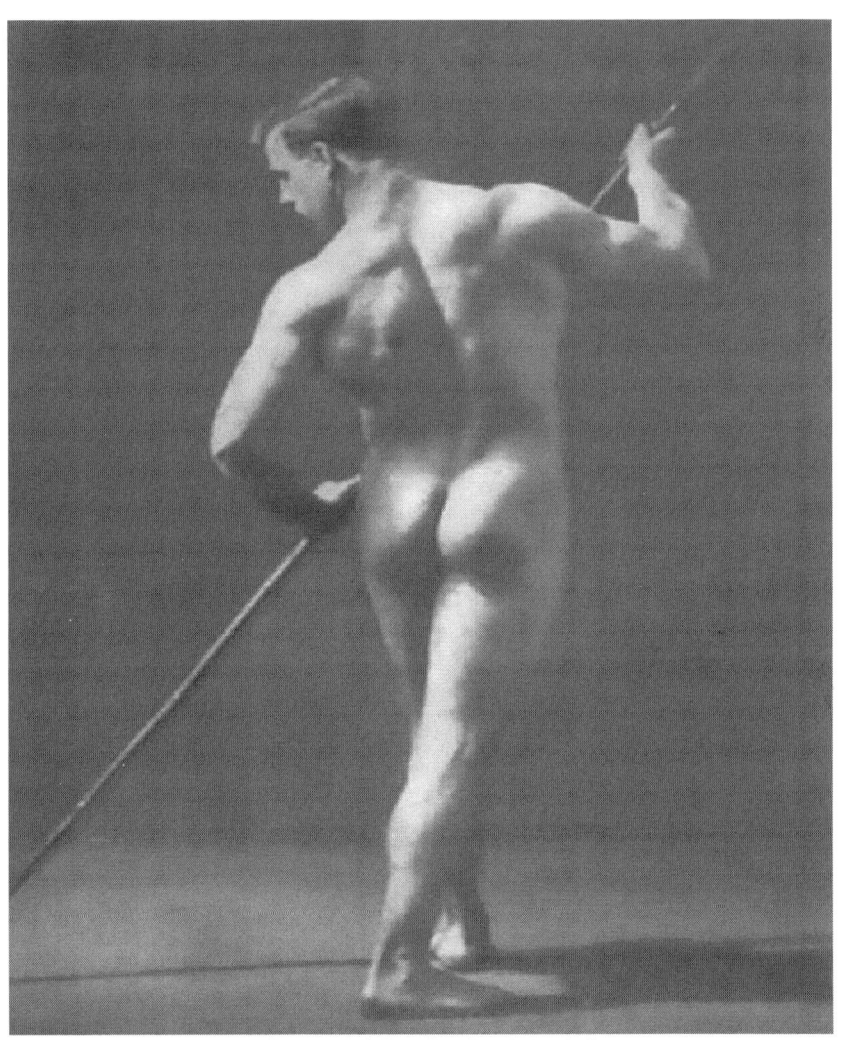

A Graceful Study: by Maxick.

HEALTH, STRENGTH & WILL-POWER THROUGH NATURAL PHYSICAL CULTURE,
by MAXICK & SALDO.

CONTENTS.

	PAGE
Brief Apology	2
Warning to Readers	2
Preface (Introduction to The Last Word in Physical Culture)	4
Maxaldo Methods	6
The Objects of our Methods	8
What the Maxick-Saldo System of P.C. is	10
The Evolution of the System	13
Muscle-Control in relation to Great Strength	15
Abdominal Control	16
The System of the Future	17
Indigestion	18
Constipation	19
An Object Lesson in Chest Development	20
A Word upon other Systems	24
Terms	27
How the Treatment is Carried out	28
The Maxaldo Muscle-Control Competition	29

MAXICK & SALDO,

Specialists in Curative, Physical Culture,

65 & 66, Piccadilly,

LONDON, W.

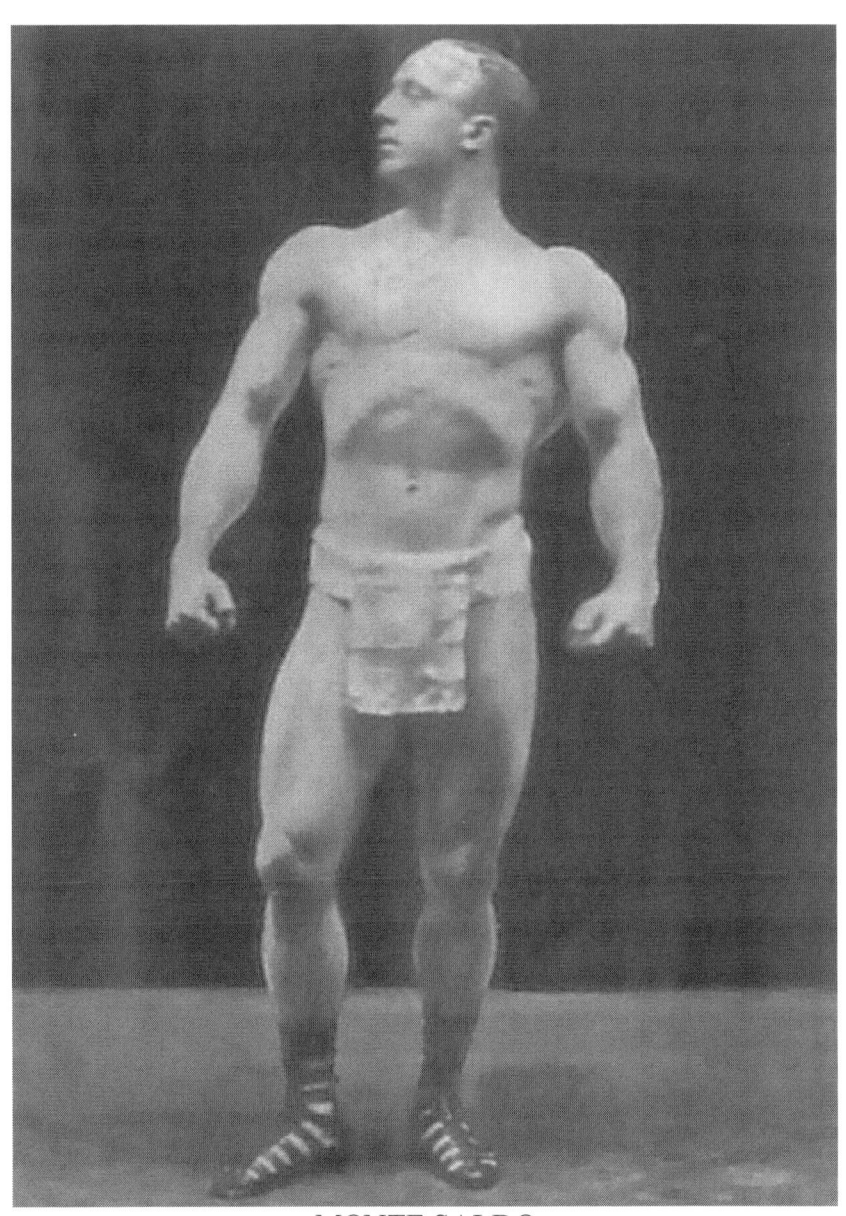
MONTE SALDO

BRIEF APOLOGY.

IN practically every explanatory booklet of a System of Physical Culture, long wearying chapters upon the advantages of the subject have to be waded through.

We lay no claim to brilliance of intellect, in having realised, that any applicant for particulars of a System, is sufficiently aware of the value of Physical Culture to render such waste of the applicant's time entirely superfluous.

Being practical men, whose time is valuable, is costs us no effort to imagine that your time may also be just as valuable, and this is our only apology for the brevity of this modest booklet.

WARNING TO READERS.

A number of small imitators spring up from time to time. Their stock-in-trade usually consists of photographs of one or two of OUR PUPILS, performing muscle-control feats (particularly the isolated abdominal control); whole paragraphs of our literature, and a lot of exaggerated claims about medals and obscure championships.

We have just had handed to us another booklet, from just such a gentleman at Plaistow, which for cool impertinence would be impossible to beat.

These fellows who try to steal others' brains, are always mentally sluggish; and their almost pathetic belief that the public are on a mental plane with themselves, would account for the manner in which they approach public notice.

HEALTH STRENGTH & WILL-POWER THROUGH NATURAL
PHYSICAL CULTURE

Superb development of the Intercostal Muscles.

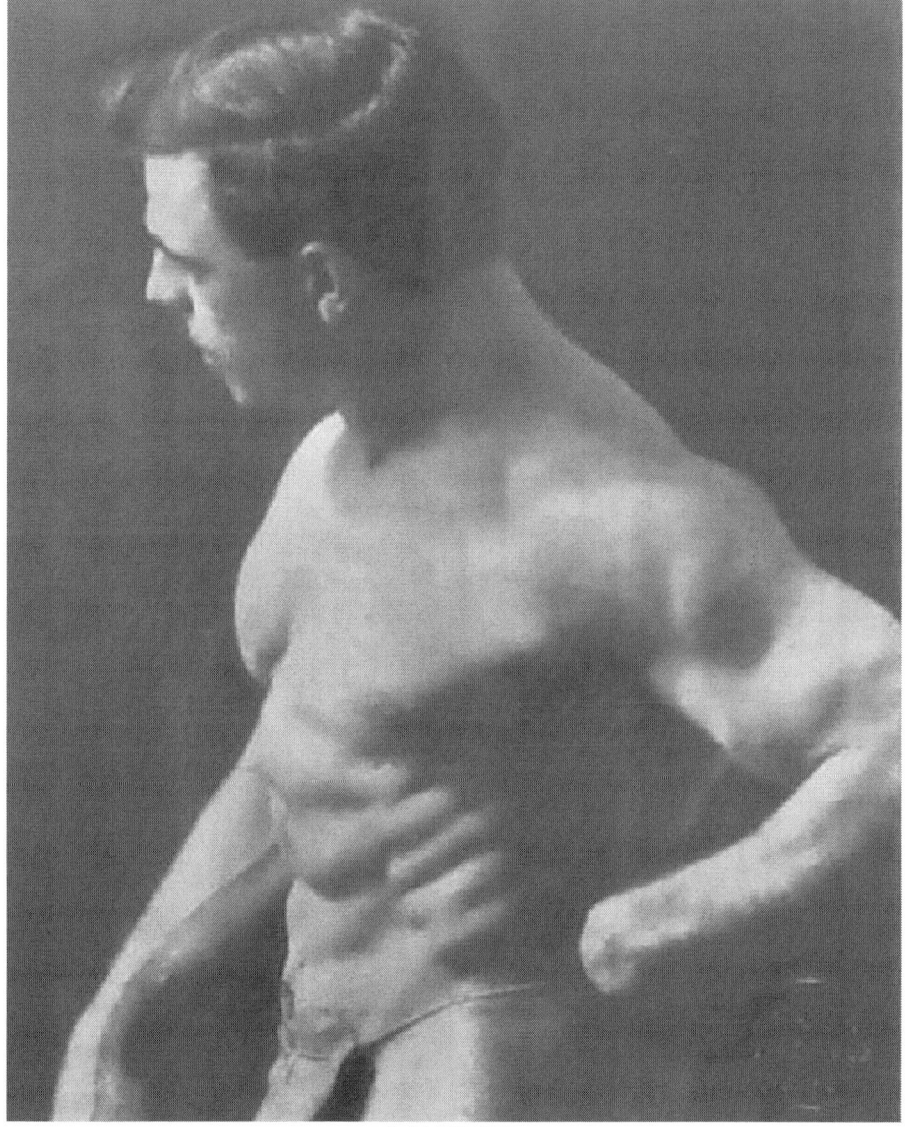

MAXICK.

THE LAST WORD IN

PHYSICAL CULTURE

PREFACE.

In presenting the revised edition of our epoch-making booklet, "The Last Word in Physical Culture," we take pleasure in assuring the public that the System to which we justly apply the above title, and which we have now been teaching for upwards of 3 years, continues to be the "Last Word."

The best cannot be improved upon, therefore the System remains unchanged; and, in view of the mutability of some systems now on the market, this fact alone should commend our methods.

We have had occasion to deal elsewhere with the Physical Culture Shark; and our present prominent position in the Physical Culture World is partly due to the fearless manner in which we have exposed their fraudulent practices.

Without recapitulation, it is sufficient to relate how a few quacks, with shameless rapacity, who spared neither the health nor pockets of their pray, cast discredit upon a profession which is amongst the most honourable. Through their abominable practices, the honour of genuine teachers had been besmirched, and the faith of the public undermined to an inestimable degree. But in the face of this, and opposed by a partial press, we set about the arduous task of winning the confidence of the public. That we have done so is proved by the support which has been extended to us from all parts of the globe. Our name has become a guarantee of probity throughout the Physical Culture World, and nothing which is not perfectly clean can be imputed to us. In all our dealings, everything has been above-board. The "fake" matches which have become a feature in many sports have never had our support, and though, more than once we have been alone in the censure of this degradation of sport, we have never failed to put the perpetrators beneath the lash. We shall not hesitate, should occasion arise, to do all in our power to eradicate this opprobrium, both from the

Sports allied to physical culture, and the Profession of Physical Culture Specialist.

Confident of the continued support of the public, we shall continue to teach the true methods by which physical perfection may be attained.

The interested perusal of the following pages will convince the layman no less than the athlete, of the efficacy of our System.

MAXALDO METHODS.

Owe their existence to the discovery of the Natural Law, which provides that certain parts of the human frame increase in size, power, and adaptability, in proportion to the use made of them. This, regarded in the abstract, is profoundly simple; but it is when we seek to apply this Law that its complexity becomes apparent. A complete knowledge of the many parts that go to make this law is essential to the Physical Culture Specialist, as well as a sense of true proportion. This sense is sadly lacking in many P.C. Specialists of to-day, as will be proved to the reader's satisfaction. In order to do this it is necessary to say that any exercises performed, or any exertion made with a view to increasing the Physical power, must not be carried far enough to induce excessive fatigue. This fact has been apparently overlooked by most teachers, whose summary advice is "to work until the muscles are incapable of doing anything further for the time being," or words to that effect. They also give their unfortunate pupils to understand that, "the more work done the more benefit gained, etc.," regardless of the physical strength, will, and capabilities of the individual.

The perils of such advice cannot be over estimated, but unfortunately is carried to even greater and more dangerous lengths, upon which we have spoken elsewhere. Here, however, it is sufficient to say that a man who advises Heavy Weight-lifting as a cure for weak heart, and as a valuable medium for increasing the height, should be avoided. There is no possible argument to back up such advice; indeed the whole of medical and physical Science is against it.

HEALTH STRENGTH & WILL-POWER THROUGH NATURAL PHYSICAL CULTURE

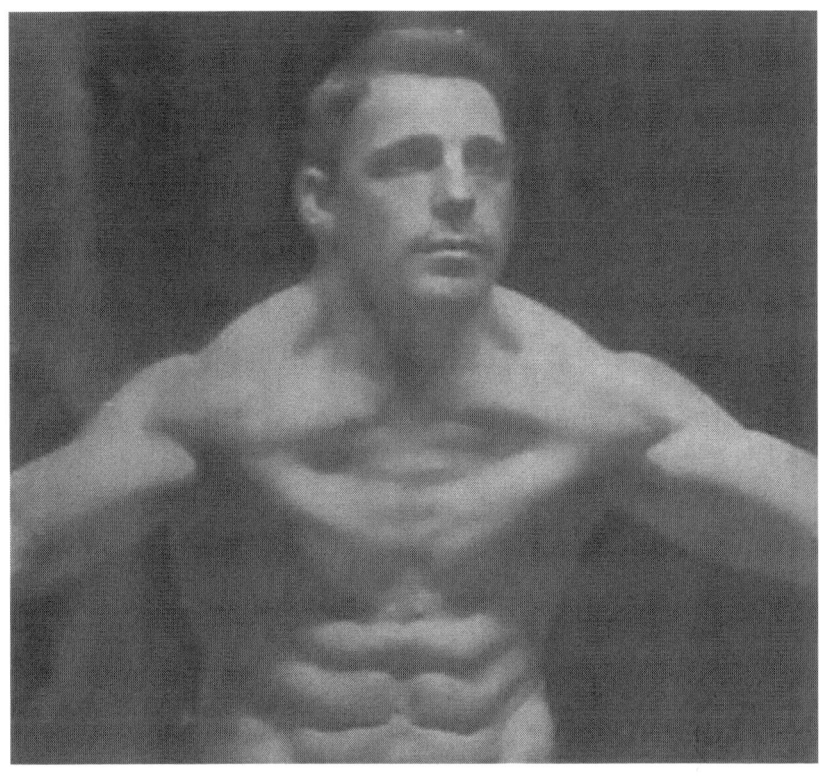

MAXICK – Holder of the following World's Weight-lifting Records, all performed in London, before members of the B.W.L.A. Committee:

Two-handed Jerk, 322 ½ lbs.   Two-handed Press, 254 lbs.
Two-handed Clean, 272 ½ lbs. One-handed Jerk, 232 ½ lbs.
                              One-handed Snatch, 162 ½ lbs.

Maxick only became a weight-lifter to prove on the scales that his method gives greater strength than any other yet known.

THE OBJECTS OF OUR METHODS.

We aim, first and foremost, at the improvement of the Circulation, it being through that channel alone that every function of the body can gain vigour, and acquire increased activity and endurance.

This is not attained by several hundreds of movements gone through daily with dumb-bells or some apparatus, nor by the tremendous output of energy which this involves. The energy must be retained and added to, and this is the end which we have in view in our System, as the whole of our teaching consists in the conserving of energy, by economizing the output; and, furthermore, in showing how to direct the energy to the best advantage.

It is not in "mad endeavour" that objects are attained, but the judicious employment of our powers, that leads to success; and upon these lines we work.

It would not be difficult to trace out the results of following a System which does not involve loss of energy, and great fatigue; but space is limited, and, moreover, we do not wish to trouble the reader to wade through the sands of Scientific Facts, which brought us to discover the most wonderful System of which we have record.

HEALTH STRENGTH & WILL-POWER THROUGH NATURAL PHYSICAL CULTURE

An Exercise of the System being illustrated by Mr. Maxick. The absolute steadiness of the photograph proves that no effort is being made to hold this contraction. It is knowing where to pull and what to press in the early stages that gives this extraordinary power and control.

P.S. – It is impossible either to secure or retain this development with apparatus or weights.

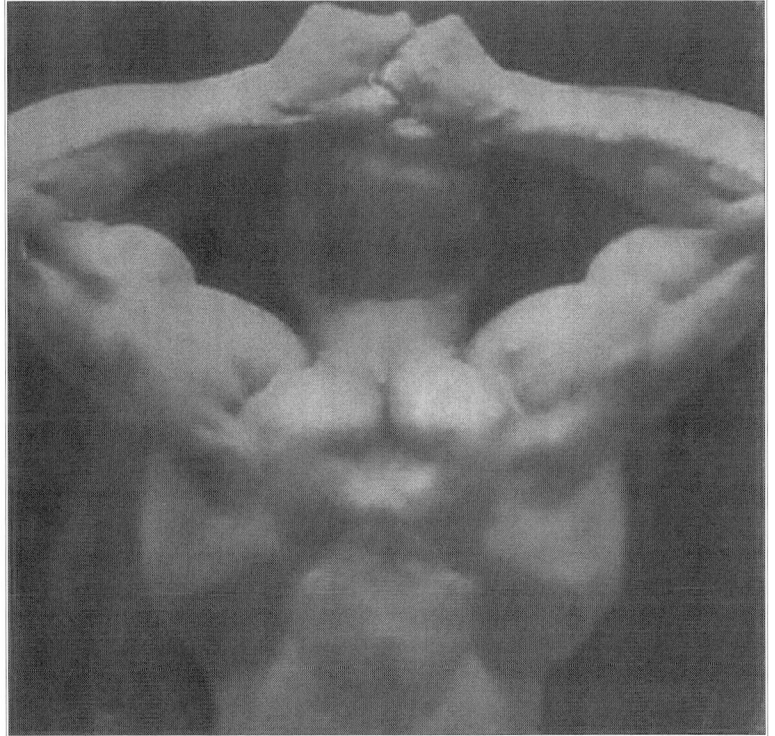

MAXICK.

A Favourite Pose of Imitators.

WHAT THE MAXICK-SALDO SYSTEM OF PHYSICAL CULTURE IS.

The System is a combination of two kinds of exercises, *i.e.*, Mechanical and Control. The Mechanical Exercises, although requiring a certain amount of energy to perform, compel the muscles to work, and thus prepare them for, and render them susceptible to, the control which constitutes the ground-work of the system.

As the concentrative power of the mind increases, the greater becomes the controlling force, and the less mechanical or energy-wasting work is required. Eventually the mechanical exercises may be left out entirely, for the proficient student will be able to thoroughly exercise all muscles, the internal as well as external layers, without any output of energy.

This enables a busy man, who has neither time nor convenience for going through an elaborate course of daily training with some of the inventions with which the market is flooded, to keep himself thoroughly fit and efficient with ten minutes daily exercise, without the inconvenience of apparatus.

Successful Musicians, Artists, and Business Men all owe their success to control.

To gain control is one of the simplest things in the world, but like many other simple things, the way to do it had to be discovered.

As the Romans, at the height of their intellectual culture, were ignorant of the first laws of hydraulics (an ignorance which caused them to build those mighty Aquaducts, some of which are almost 70 miles in length), so is the ordinary Physical Culturist lacking in knowledge of the simplest laws through whose agency strength and fitness are obtained. He goes the longest way round because he has had no opportunity of knowing better. If he gets anywhere eventually, it is greatly to his credit, because he has, no doubt, had to face many set-backs, and has, probably, handed out a lot of money into the bargain.

To resume, control teaches you where to pull and where to

press; using the various salient points of the bone as fulcra, and the muscles and joints as levers. Even the tendons become plastic and pliable, and will lose the toughness which many years' wrong exercising has caused.

Even the air pressure is used to assist in a certain relaxed contraction. (See photos of Abdominal Control of Maxick, Saldo and pupils).

Then comes the awakening of a sympathy between the brain and the muscles, which is marked in the beginning, by a greater clearness of mental power, and increased responsive power on the part of the muscles. Then as the circulation of the blood, the organs of digestion, elimination and respiration become subjective to the will, you have gained the power of keeping absolutely healthy and fit, without any inconvenience or apparatus.

You cannot possibly become stale or tired, as is the inevitable result of training with bells or chest expanders.

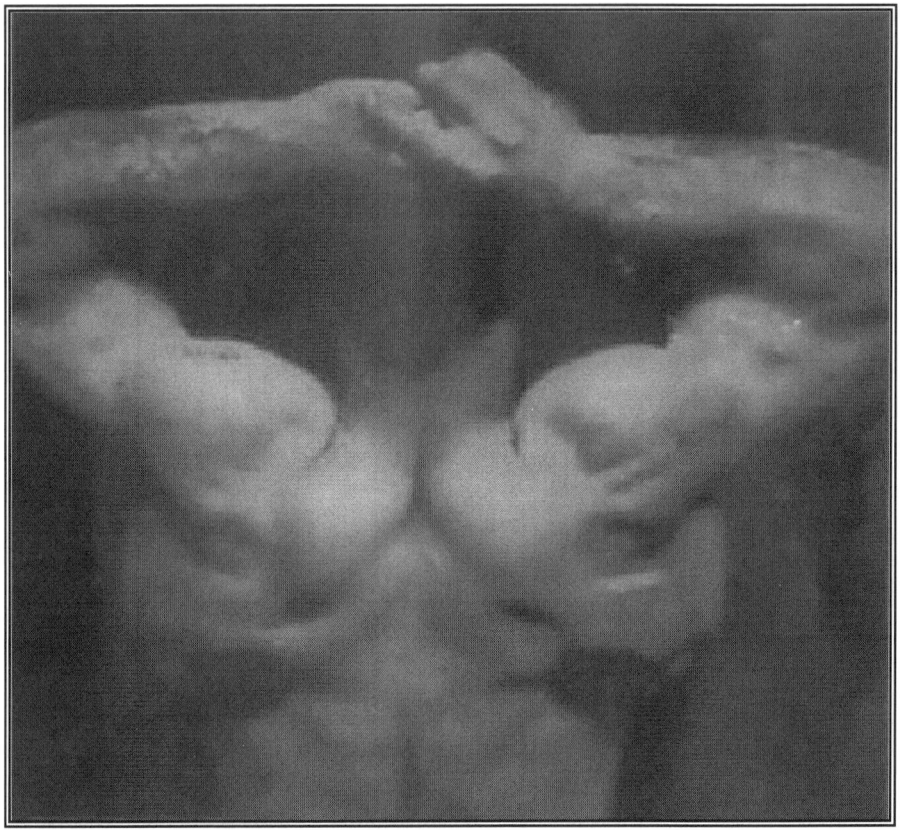

SALDO – The only Light-weight man in England holding British Heavyweight Records, which are:

Left-handed Clean, 202 ½lbs.   Left-handed Snatch, 154lbs.

He also performed the Single-handed Clean World's Record of 212 lbs. with the right hand at 10st. 7lbs. and was the first man in the world to swing to arm's length above head, a weight much heavier than himself.

THE EVOLUTION OF THE SYSTEM.

The Maxick-Saldo System of Physical Culture is the outcome of years of practical study, research, and experiment, and is **not** a free-movement System.

Being based upon the latest discoveries in physiological and psychological science it admits an element unknown in any other System, *i.e.*, the Mind. The application of the subjective mental faculties, which is essential to the attainment of any mental knowledge whatsoever, is equally necessary whether improvement of the Physique, the acquisition of Health, or increase in Strength be desired.

It is the only System wherein the individuality of the pupil is permitted to have any part. The absence of other apparatus than the mind assures this. The mind directs the effort, and according to the quality of the motive force, so the Physical improvement is determined.

The strongest part of a man is his individuality; and instead of allowing him to subjugate this by advising the employment of external apparatus, we assist him to use this power to the attainment of the Physical condition he desires.

By studying his case, we are enabled to judge of his adaptability to apply himself to the task in hand, and to direct these powers to his own good. At the same time we can ascertain wherein lies, not only his Physical, but his Mental lack of Control.

By a carefully graduated series of exercises, most of which cannot be performed without diligent application of the mind, we bring out the best powers of the mental and physical functions.

At the same time, by careful advice regarding diet, bathing, and other matters of hygiene, we bring these powers into a state of perfection.

Anything to which we apply the activity of our minds is bound to have more substantial, durable and far-reaching effects upon us, than that which comes to us unsought, and which we accept passively.

The effort expended in the attainment of any mental or physical good has in itself built up a power which mere passivity will never achieve. Therefore our System is pre-eminently the one to be chosen by the intending student, inasmuch as genuine efforts must be put forth to learn the exercises.

Among the many great advantages, which would take many pages to explain effectually – on account of their relation to the psychological elements of our existence – the absence of monotony should commend itself most forcibly. Nature's antipathy to monotony, depicted in the variety of all around us, is no less strongly established in the mind of man; and this fact has not been forgotten in building up our System. The many who turn to Physical Culture as a recreation and a relaxation from the exigencies and turmoil of modern life make this a necessity; for it is essential that there be an interest, apart from the physical exertion involved; something which would call forth other powers of the mind than those used in carrying out the daily duties. It is in this gradual drawing out of various branches of the mind, which the correct performance of the exercises necessitates, the sense of time, of posture, and many other qualities, that this recreation finds place. True recreation should help one in the work of the day, by storing up a plenitude of physical and mental energy, and this is what we claim a treatment under us will accomplish.

MUSCLE-CONTROL IN RELATION TO GREAT STRENGTH.

In reply to those who would ask whether Muscle-control gives great strength, we would reply, that the two most important strength matches of modern times were won by the men we backed and trained.

As a further proof that muscles produced by this most Natural Method will give greater energy and Strength than that produced by lifting, Maxick issues the following challenge: –

"I will match myself to lift against any man in the world, weight for weight on pure strength lifts. I will even reduce my weight to 9 stone 7 lbs. to meet a man of that weight if he does not care to take advantage of the weight for weight offer.

Further I will undertake not to indulge in any exercise with weights or to practice with bars of any description for at least three months before the test if desired by my opponent.

Full facilities will be given to any opponent to enable him to be thoroughly satisfied that the conditions are carried out to the letter."

Note. – **MAXICK & SALDO**, although taking no active interest in Weight-lifting, **HOLD PRACTICALLY ALL THE WORLD'S STRENGTH RECORDS** between them.

ABDOMINAL CONTROL.

The Value of Abdominal Control from a Health standpoint, cannot be over-estimated. Without resorting to Pseudo Physiological terms, we will, in as simple a manner as possible, explain the reasons. To possess the power of lifting the relaxed abdominal wall at will, and contracting it in any position, either horizontally or perpendicularly (without going so far as to accomplish the "one-sided" abdominal contraction feat) means that you have a perfect massage of the stomach and intestines always at hand. What are the direct result? (1) The ejection of all matter from the intestines; (2) A sufficient flow of gastric juice in the stomach follows automatically.

MAXICK is the **Discoverer** of the **"Isolated Abdominal Control,"** of which Photographs have appeared from time to time in the Magazines.

Unsolicited testimonials from all parts of the world prove that **Chronic Indigestion, Constipation,** and Stomach **Disorders** have been **absolutely eradicated** by means of a special treatment, including the secrets of Abdominal Control, in a few weeks, when all other remedies and mechanical exercises had failed.

THE SYSTEM OF THE FUTURE.

We know that with certain modifications, our System is the System of the future; and although we do not get the credit, other teachers are using our methods of training to produce excellent pupils for advertising purposes, in order to enable them to sell their old-fashioned goods.

We have only one System, and trade under one name only.

We do not use machine duplicated letters of advice in conducting a pupil's case.

We do not pester you with "follow ups."

We have seen the impossibility of dealing separately in this booklet with all the complaints and health troubles that come before us from time to time.

The cost of such a publication would entail considerably more expense to the pupil; and then it could only deal in generalities, which are useless where individual complaints and peculiarities are concerned.

It is for that reason therefore that we request you to give us particulars upon the form that accompanies this book, which will enable us to make a diagnosis of your case, as suggested on page 28.

Two Short Articles, dealing with Indigestion and Constipation, appear on pages 18 and 19.

INDIGESTION.

It is generally understood that the digestive process, from the act of swallowing to defecation is entirely dependent upon certain reflex nervous actions. Most of the specialists whose systems we have perused seem ignorant of the fact that the outflow of saliva, of gastric juice and bile (to mention a few of the better known of the many more or less complicated chemical compounds that encounter the food in its passage through the digestive tract) is due to and controlled by action of the nervous System.

To fully understand this important fact, it is only necessary to realize that the outflow of the various juices necessary to digestion, are capable of being inhibited by certain emotional states, an ever apparent instance being the cessation of the flow of saliva which causes dryness of the mouth when in a state of fear or anger.

Our remarkable success in the treatment of digestive disturbances is due in no small measure to our recognition of the above important facts, as well as to our methods of treating Indigestion, not as a complaint in itself, but as the result of one or more of many contributory causes. At the same time we are not oblivious of the fact that Indigestion may in its turn contribute to pathological conditions of far greater seriousness.

Another great asset which we are able to bring to the treatment of this and other disorders is our knowledge of curative treatments required under all kinds of climatic conditions. Our studies have been pursued in many parts of the world, and we have treated successfully under circumstances of the greatest difficulty, owing to the impossibility of obtaining suitable articles of diet, and the consequent inability to use dietic precautions. Under such conditions we have had to employ the most careful treatment, and we claim that this international and world-wide experience has given us the power and ability to treat digestive and allied disorders with greater success than any other specialists extant.

CONSTIPATION.

Although Constipation is attributed to many causes, it is most frequently due to lack of muscular tone in the intestines, and the consequent relaxed condition of the intestinal wall; or an imperfect or deficient secretion of the intestinal fluids. The existence of these conditions however may be traced chiefly to the habit of taking Drugs.

The ill-consequences of Constipation are so many, that it would be impossible to outline them here; but it is sufficiently obvious that the absorption of poisons into the blood-stream which results from the retention of waste matter in the intestine must be fraught with grave dangers to health; and piles, indigestion, flatulence, nervous disorders, furred tongue, lassitude, are a few of the many serious ailments which may result from faulty elimination.

The action of drugs seldom prevents these resultant effects of Constipation, for the contents of the intestine do not move steadily, but remain stationary until the drug liquify the already fermented and morbid matter, and passes it suddenly.

Having realised that a real and permanent cure for constipation would mean all the difference between Good Health and Bad Health to a considerable proportion of the world's inhabitants, we made careful experiments, and before we began teaching publicly, five years ago, had so perfected our methods, that not in any single case handled by us, have we failed to permanently eradicate this really appalling disorder.

Any cases accepted by us for eradication are strictly under guarantee.

MAXICK is here shown in an object lesson in Chest Development.

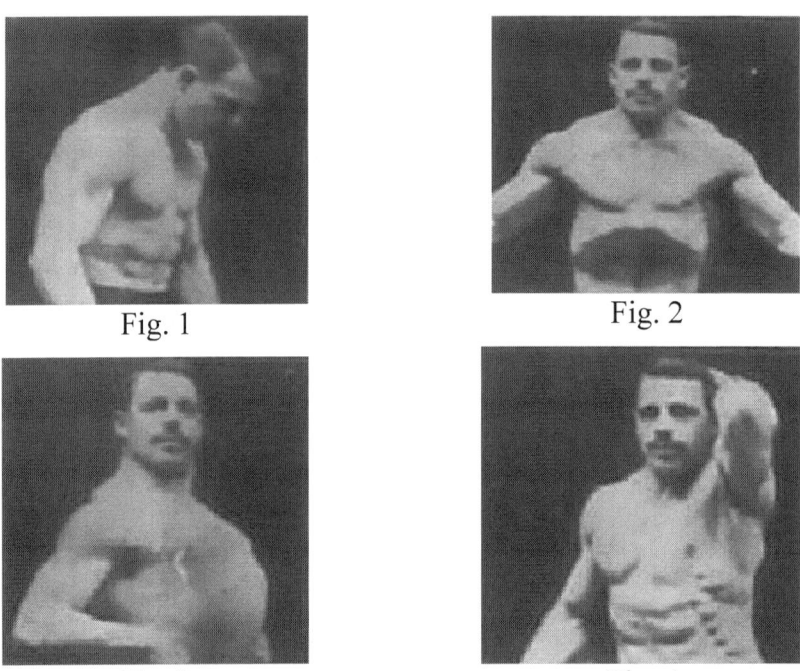

Fig. 1

Fig. 2

Fig. 3

Fig. 4

Fig. 1 – Unconscious and dangerous attitude taken up by the average man.

Fig. 2 – Correct method of holding the chest up, without the assistance of the lungs.

Fig. 3 – Incorrect method of holding the chest up, by filling the lungs with air. As soon as the air is expelled, the chest drops to position 1.

Fig. 4 – Development of the Abdominal and Intercostal (between rib) Muscles only possible by our methods.

> It is these muscles that keep the chest lifted, and allow the lungs free play, but they must be full and supple, correctly filling the intervals between the ribs.

HEALTH STRENGTH & WILL-POWER THROUGH NATURAL PHYSICAL CULTURE

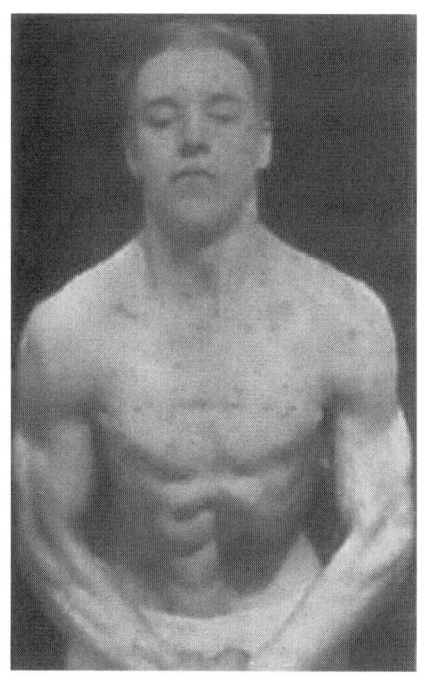

RITCHIE, BIRMINGHAM.

Superb expositions of the isolated abdominal control,

performed by

Mr. A. W. BEETON

(top photograph)

and

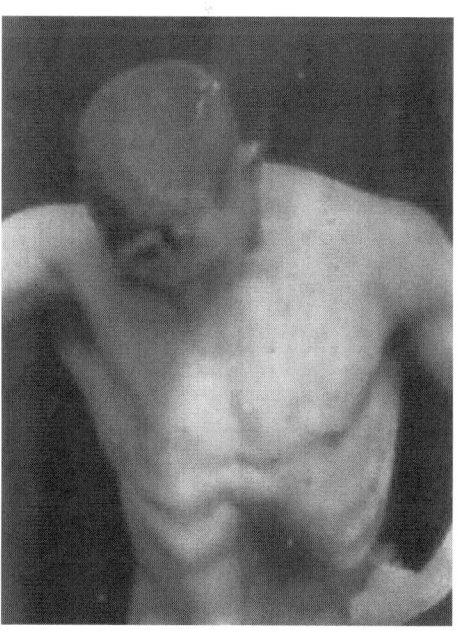

JOSEPH LILLY

(lower photograph)

Mr. Beeton was instructed-by mail in England; and

Mr. Lilly by mail at Gibraltar.

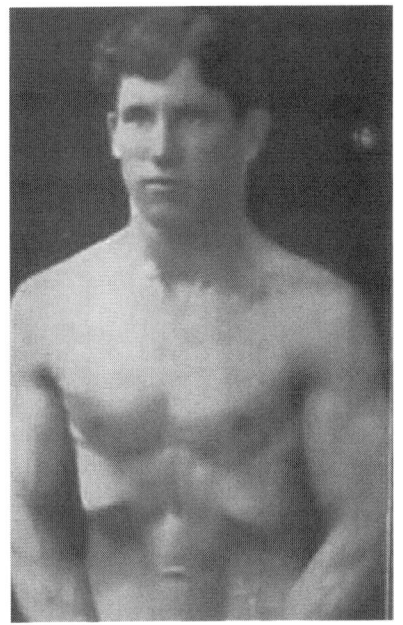

Two fine examples of the central isolation of the abdominal muscles, performed by

BERT GRAHAM

(top photo.)

and

DAVID BLAZER

(lower photo.)

Mr. Graham resides in Australia, and was instructed by mail.

Mr. Blazer was instructed by mail when touring in the Tropics.

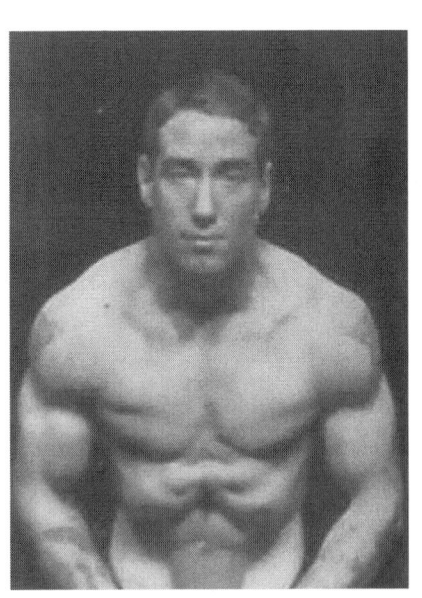

The above Feat is a Favourite of our Imitators.

HEALTH STRENGTH & WILL-POWER THROUGH NATURAL
PHYSICAL CULTURE

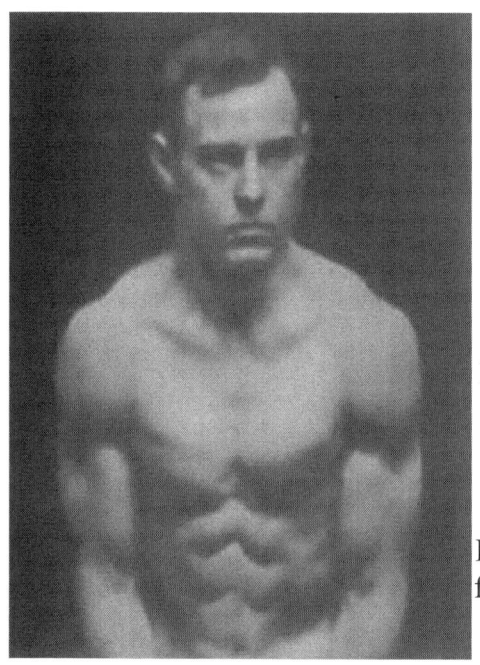

Pupil ALBERT SOGUEL

(top photo).

9st. 7lbs. Weight-lifting Champion of the World.

Soguel performed the unheard of feat of snatching, in one clean movement from floor to above head with one hand.

144 ½lbs.; 12 ½lbs, more than his own weight!

This lift is one that requires tremendous energy.

He holds the B.W.L.A. Certificate for the above feat, and also for the Single-handed Clean Lift of 182½lbs., both World's Records.

Pupil – JOSEPH WÜHR

(lower photo)

One of the four men in the world who have succeeded in raising more than double their own body-weight above head in a double-handed jerk.

Mr. Wühr is here shown contracting the muscles of the Abdomen perpendicularly.

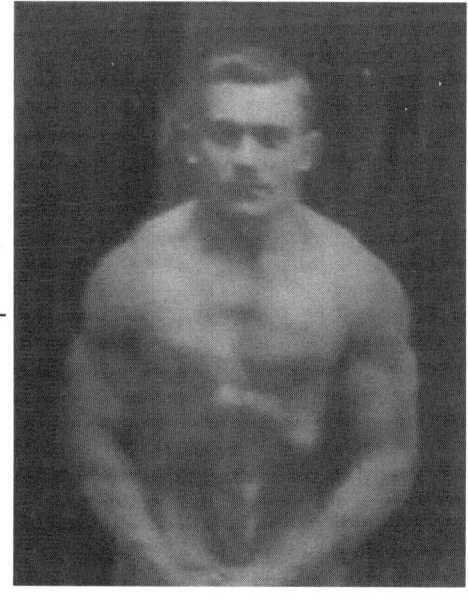

A WORD UPON OTHER SYSTEMS.

THERE are many of these on the market at present; some good, some indifferent, and others bad.

The whole Physical Culture World was highly entertained recently by the appearance of an advertisement in which the inventor assured the public that there was *no* fear of his system producing big muscles. He has not done much advertising since; the reasons doubtless being that the public realized at once that a system that would not produce big muscles, would not produce small ones; and that such a system would be useless.

For you cannot even digest a cherry without the action of several internal muscle groups. Further, in spite of the cry of the attenuated P.C. Specialist, "My System will not produce muscular development," it is the desire of most men to possess a pleasing and symmetrical body as well as Good Health. It is by no means necessary for a healthy man to be of the angular and knotted-knee variety.

Great amusement has been caused lately by the claim of a P.C. Teacher that he has no System; and he continues in the vein that all Systems are dangerous, cut-and-dried, useless, etc. It may of course be a feeble attempt at originality, but we should be pleased to know, from what then does this gentleman select suitable exercises for his pupils, if he has not a complete system? Surely he does not invent new exercises for each pupil, and prescribe them, without first making experiments of each exercise, covering long periods, to prove the efficacy and safety of such exercises!

For the maintenance of good health big muscles are not necessary; in fact they are, in a way, a drain upon the vitality of the subject if produced by forced, unnatural means. It is the invisible muscles that work the processes of digestion, and it is to these that we give the greatest attention.

When it comes to chest development however, the visible muscles require attention; for, as the following illustration, on page 20, will explain, a permanent development of chest cannot be gained from breathing exercises alone. The muscles between the ribs require correctly developing.

Mere bending and joint movements only just tend to keep one fairly fit; and the energy that is thus expended, with practically no benefit except to the circulation, might have been used in building the body up to good proportions, a thing of which no man need be ashamed.

The Spartan-like treatment to which so many seekers after a better condition of health subject themselves is little short of madness. The idea of exercising in winter, before an open window, with little or no clothing is one of the most pernicious of the many that have unfortunately taken root in the world of Physical Culture.

Cold is life's greatest enemy. If one exercise in a cold room, energy and vitality are being used up all the time to keep the body warm. The object of exercise is to get the blood to the different parts of the body, to nourish them. Why, then, go to the trouble to exercise at all if you are going to expose the body to the cold and so drive the blood from the parts needing it. You will usually find that the followers of such systems have thin tough muscles, whereas a healthy, properly nourished muscle should be full, round and supple.

We find that a large number of people who have followed Physical Culture for a year or two, are most terribly muscle-bound. When they try to lift the chest, they feel a tightness around the ribs, while the shoulder blades appear to be cemented to the sides.

They are also usually unable to relax the muscles of the abdomen correctly. To contract the most easily controlled muscle on the body, *i.e.*, the muscles of the upper arm, they usually have to clench the fist. It is a chronic state of hardness that the muscles have been brought to by continued contraction, without correct relaxation, stretching and control.

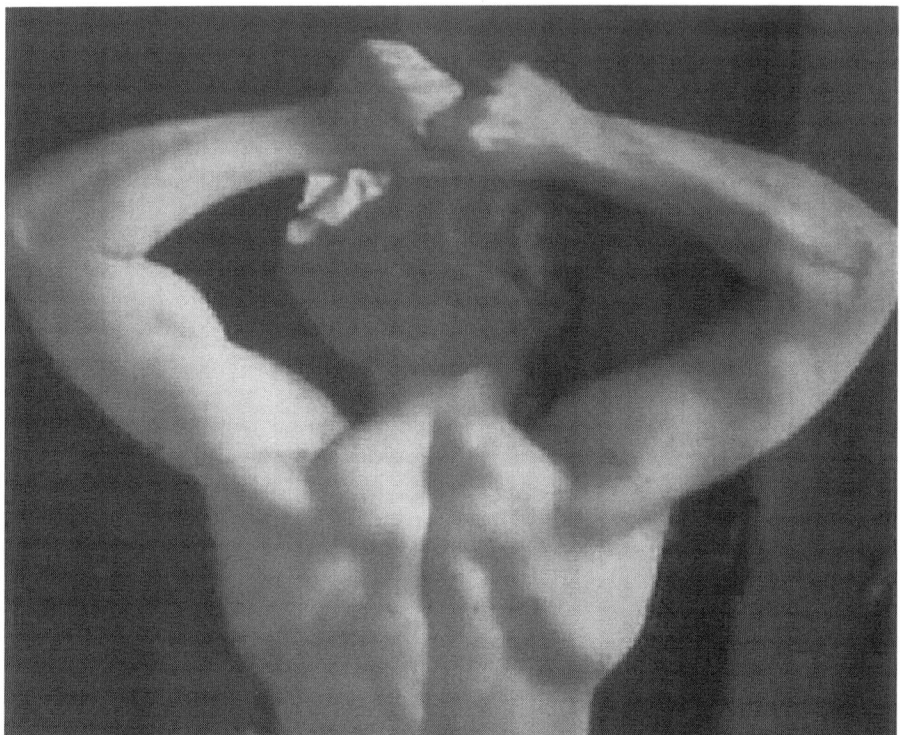

ATHELDA - This photograph of an Englishwoman, trained to this marvelous pitch speaks eloquently for our methods. There is none of the stringiness usually found in ladies who have used Chest-expanders and Dumb-bells, but full, healthy, massive muscles.

This lady holds the Maxick-Saldo Golden Award for Muscle-Control, and is far stronger than the average man.

P.S. – These muscles, when in repose, form a smooth, supple surface, all traces of the individual muscles disappearing.

TERMS.

The cost of treatment will naturally depend upon the ailment treated, and the duration of the course. Upon receiving particulars of the case from the prospective pupil, we shall be able to give definite information upon this matter. Our fees are extremely moderate, and are arranged on strictly practical lines.

The exorbitant charges asked by some Physical Culture teachers and the subsequent reduction, often down to a few shillings, are nothing less than a scandal, and only prove that if you had paid the first fee asked, you would have been well fleeced.

For an all-round increase in fitness and general muscular development, a course of six lessons is prescribed. Unless otherwise arranged, these are sent at fortnightly intervals; the inclusive fee being, £2 2s. 0d.

HOW THE TREATMENT OF THE TWO-GUINEA COURSE IS CARRIED OUT.

(1) Particulars received from prospective pupil.

(2) The case is studied and the diagnosis is returned to the pupil. If we are able to undertake the case, any extra particulars required of the pupil are asked, and we are then prepared to treat.

(3) The first section of exercises is sent. Included is a special letter of advice, treating all points, and comprehending diet, bathing, etc., taking into strict consideration the particular requirements, age and profession of the pupil.

(4) From time to time during the Course we receive reports of the progress that is being made, which enables us to treat with even greater precision, both as regards advice and the prescription of suitable exercises.

The remaining lessons are sent at pre-arranged intervals, or may be prolonged or sent at even shorter intervals, as directed by the pupil.

In this Course, when considered necessary, or desired by pupil, the control of the muscles is taught as depicted in the photographs of pupils on pages 21, 22 and 23.

In all cases installments may be arranged to suit the pupil's convenience.

HEALTH STRENGTH & WILL-POWER THROUGH NATURAL PHYSICAL CULTURE

THE MAXALDO MUSCLE-CONTROL COMPETITION.

MAXICK & SALDO hold an Annual

"MUSCLE-CONTROL"

COMPETITION,

and present Five Gold, Twenty Silver and Fifty Bronze Medals to the 75 pupils who show, in order of merit, the nearest development to Maxick, in any of the poses contained in their system, by the 31st December, of any year. To pupils residing in the Colonies or abroad, four weeks longer will be allowed.

No pupil having won our Gold Medal will be allowed to compete again.

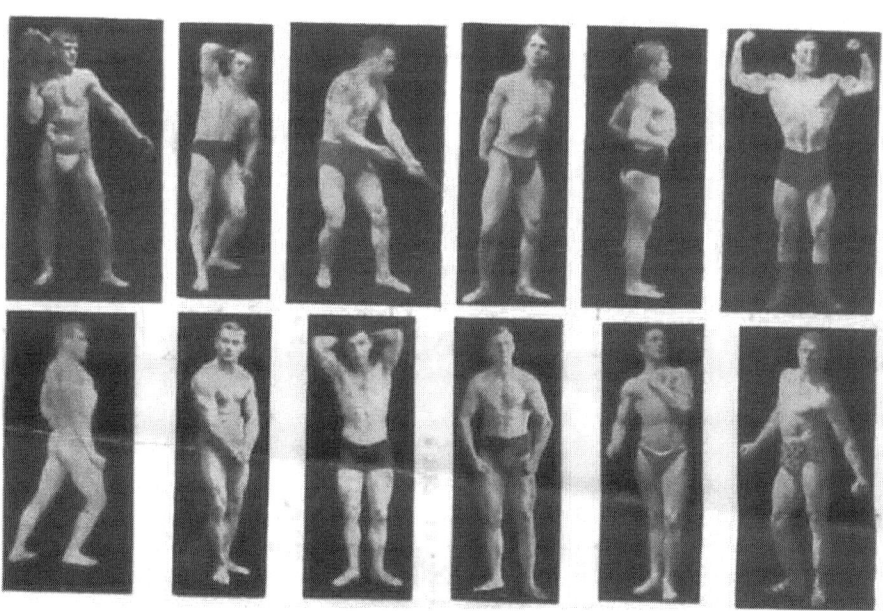

12 MAIL-INSTRUCTED PUPILS

For more old time classics of strength, visit:

STRONGMANBOOKS.COM

Title Currently Available from Authors Including:
Arthur Saxon

Maxick

George F. Jowett

Otto Arco

Eugene Sandow

Bob Hoffman and the York Company

George Hackenschmidt

Edward Aston

and more...

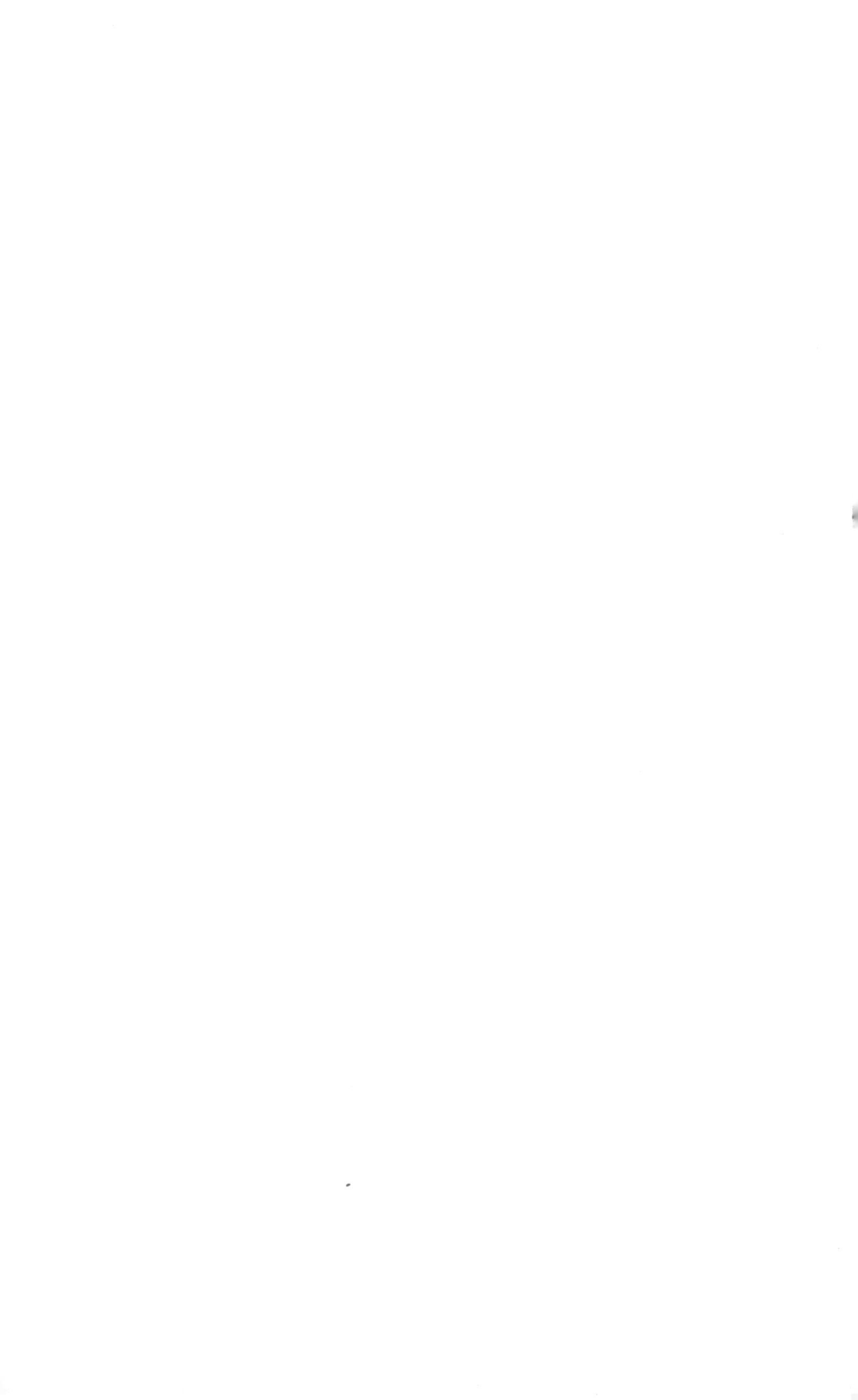

Made in the USA
Monee, IL
18 October 2021